BODYBUILDING

Building the Perfect Body With Simple Hints and Tips for Beginners Lose Fitness Training

(The Formula of Hypertrophy Optimize Training Nutrition to Stimulate Maximal Muscle Growth)

Jose Perry

Published By John Kembrey

Jose Perry

All Rights Reserved

Body Building: Building the Perfect Body With Simple Hints and Tips for Beginners Lose Fitness Training (The Formula of Hypertrophy Optimize Training Nutrition to Stimulate Maximal Muscle Growth)

ISBN 978-1-77485-355-9

All rights reserved. No part of this guide may be reproduced in any form without permission in writing from the publisher except in the case of brief quotations embodied in critical articles or reviews.

Legal & Disclaimer

The information contained in this book is not designed to replace or take the place of any form of medicine or professional medical advice. The information in this book has been provided for educational and entertainment purposes only.

The information contained in this book has been compiled from sources deemed reliable, and it is accurate to the best of the Author's knowledge; however, the Author cannot guarantee its accuracy and validity and cannot be held liable for any errors or omissions. Changes are periodically made to this book. You must consult your doctor or get professional medical advice before using any of the suggested remedies, techniques, or information in this book.

Upon using the information contained in this book, you agree to hold harmless the Author from and against any damages, costs, and expenses, including any legal fees potentially resulting from the application of any of the information provided by this guide. This disclaimer applies to any damages or injury caused by the use and application, whether directly or indirectly, of any advice or information presented, whether for breach of contract, tort, negligence, personal injury, criminal intent, or under any other cause of action.

You agree to accept all risks of using the information presented inside this book. You need to consult a professional medical practitioner in order to ensure you are both able and healthy enough to participate in this program.

TABLE OF CONTENTS

INTRODUCTION 1

CHAPTER 1: HORMONES, HORMONES, HORMONES 5

CHAPTER 2: NUTRITION 35

CHAPTER 3: WORKOUT PLANS 45

CHAPTER 4: WHY IT IS IMPORTANT TO BUILD MUSCLE 63

CHAPTER 5: THE BASIC TRAINING PRINCIPLES 73

CHAPTER 6: TRAINING AND EXERCISE EQUIPMENT 80

CHAPTER 7: TWO STEP PROCESS 94

CHAPTER 8: BENEFITS OF CARBOHYDRATES FOR BODYBUILDING 101

CHAPTER 9: ANDARINE S4 112

CHAPTER 10: WHAT IS THE THE BEST DIET FOR MUSCLES BUILDING? 124

CHAPTER 11: VEGAN BODYBUILDING MISTAKES 134

CHAPTER 12: BODYBUILDING FOR BEGINNERS 156

CHAPTER 13: HOW OFTEN EACH BODY PART IS TRAINED 164

CONCLUSION 178

Introduction

The popularity of fitness first exploded in the 1980s, when people began to understand the importance of being healthy. A huge amount of money was each year by both people and institutions to improve their fitness. Everybody was looking for the ideal body. Nowadays, gyms are found all over. Personal trainers earn their living by helping people keep healthy and fit. The supplements for bodybuilding have been gaining popularity recently and are now thought to be the "shortcut" to fitness.

In reality, bodybuilding has been in existence for a long time. Eugen Sandow, who is also known as the founder of bodybuilding in the modern age, used to allow spectators to watch his physique in various muscle-showing actions. Eugen's performances were performed during the last decade of the 20th century. He is considered to be the inventor of bodybuilding as a sports.

Eugen Sandow's shows were built on the demonstration the strength, agility and strength in order to display his impeccable body, which was at the time, believed to be the "dream" body. Sandow became so popular in the stunts he performed that he developed an entire industry around bodybuilding. Sandow was among the first to sell (and develop) products for bodybuilding and fitness equipment.

Sandow is also known for hosting the very first bodybuilding competition, dubbed"the "Great Competition" that was which was held in London. The contest is widely believed to be the foundation of other competitions like Mr. Olympia (currently the most popular bodybuilding competition around the globe).

But, it wasn't until World War II until men recognized the power of bodybuilding. In the course of war, people were encouraged to work on their physiques to get stronger and more powerful. The focus was on nutrition, the training methods were improved and equipment for bodybuilding was created to help strengthen muscles like never before. This was the time in time when the first bodybuilding associations and gyms were established. Examples of these organizations include the International Federation of Body Building and the Amateur Athletic Union.

Nearly three decades later Arnold Schwarzenegger raised the standards for men through his film "Pumping iron". Bodybuilding has now be a fad for many people all over the world. It's not just men, women too are becoming interested in the sport. The bodybuilding sport has grown into an athletic competition for women and men.

Nowadays, everyone's goal is to have the physique that was created by such athletes as Eugen Sandow, and Arnold Schwarzenneger. If you've had an interest in bodybuilding and would like to attain that 'Grecian ideal which was first thought of by Eugen Sandow This book can help you. From the basics of bodybuilding to the best way to learn the art of bodybuilding This book has all the details you require to build the ideal body.

Chapter 1: Hormones, Hormones, Hormones

Prior to anything else, you must understand how your body works prior to beginning any type of exercise. Knowing the signals your body sends will enable you to understand the need for any particular diet to improve your performance. Let's begin with hormones. Hormones play a role in every aspect of what happens, including muscle growth as well as overall health. It isn't logical to neglect your health. Being unwell results in less energy, less willpower, and a low self-esteem. There aren't the motivational factors that will help you reach your desired goal.

How do hormones work? Why are they so important to your body and your health? What ones should you be looking out for? What would happen if you had more or less? What can you do to boost hormones naturally? These questions are all answered without getting too deep into the physiology of things. This book is streamlined and simple to comprehend with even simpler methods to follow.

Changes in Mind and Body The hormones

It is well-known that exercising and healthy eating is essential to how you look and feel. Hormones affect our lives from every angle. It influences metabolism and body, as well as appetite. the weight you are carrying as well as the amount of muscle and fat you've got and affects your the level of energy, mood and mood.

When everything is in balance the metabolism will improve as will energy. This is the reason people who have a rapid and healthy metabolism are able to burn calories more effectively. The ones who have a slower metabolisms show more fat around the hips or stomach. The faster you burn calories means that you will have more energy levels which are essential to have a productive day.

There are numerous hormones, and they all play a role in a system. because I'm not here to impart knowledge about biology, I'm going explain the different hormones which affect your body's muscles, weight and overall health.

How do hormones affect you?

Specific cells release hormones which affect other cells within the body. Organs of all kinds produce hormones, and they are released into circulation of blood as well as other fluids of the body. The hormones that we create are influenced by the foods we consume and the way that we lead. Knowing which hormones have the greatest impact on the growth of muscles and weight, as well as understanding the food that affects them can help you succeed in bodybuilding, as well as any other kind of exercise you may choose to do.

You may at first be a bit surprised that I been focusing on hormones as my main priority. However they are vital. They're focused on losing fat, muscle growth and general health. It is vital to understand all there is to know regarding hormones to transform your body.

There are two kinds of hormones, anabolic and catabolic. Anabolic hormones build up the body, while the catabolic degrades the body. In the bodybuilding world this refers to anabolic hormones that aid in the development of muscles while catabolic is the reverse, which is muscle loss.

These will be the hormones sic which play the major role in muscle development as well as fat reduction. I'll discuss their role and, more importantly how you can use these hormones to improve the performance of your workout:

Testosterone

GH - growth hormone

Insulin

Thyroid hormone

Cortisol

Estrogen

Testosterone

Testosterone is also known for its role as the hormone of men due to the fact that it is responsible for male characteristics. Both men and women are affected by this hormone but in different amounts. Men possess a greater amount. It plays a vital function in the body for sexual and bodily development, metabolic and behavioral features, and more.

The male hormone is made by the testes as well as those glands that produce adrenal hormones. Once it is released into blood, around 97% of it is bound to albumin and globulin (proteins).

This binding serves three functions:

It is an storage facility or reservoir that is used to dispose of plasma fluctuations testosterone.

It shields testosterone from the liver and kidneys from degrading.

Testosterone is soluble and it is easily transported through blood.

The rest of the testosterone is not bound to plasma and hence is referred to as free testosterone. It interacts with cells and triggers physical changes.

When it comes to the regulation of T levels, it's controlled by two elements that are the binding capacity as well as the total T levels present in the blood. In other words, as the capacity to bind is increased as well as the free testosterone levels decrease. This is the reason why some T supplements and some drugs may reduce the capacity and result in freer testosterone.

When we were embryos, testosterone levels were the final say on us whether we were female or male. The testosterone production in males is present for about ten weeks after birth . When puberty begins then it ceases. It is at this point that testosterone levels are on the sky. In this phase, men display a remarkable difference to women when looking at various angles , such as the weight of their bodies and muscle structure which draws them to more intense sports such as football. It's sad that testosterone begins to diminish after the age of 30 and, by the time you reach 70-80, a third of it has disappeared.

Here's how testosterone can make everything:

The growth of the testes, scrotum and penis at puberty

The voice box is enlarged - - larynx-- and the result is more pronounced voice

The formation of sperm

Hair growth on the pubic, chest, face region (and for some guys, the back)

The skin's thickness and darkness are increased.

Sex drive increased

A higher metabolic rate

The volume of blood increases and the amount of red blood cells

Kidneys store sodium and water.

The increase in muscle protein signifies that the muscle mass is increasing

Muscle glycogen gets broken down less during exercise

Bones retain calcium

Sebaceous glands (sweat) are more active and can cause acne.

Helps to strengthen and reduce the size of the pelvis.

These are only the most prominent testosterone functions. There are numerous other effects on the body that are not included in this article. Now, I want to provide you with information about the impact of testosterone in bodybuilding.

Low Testosterone

Because testosterone is involved in many functions, if it decreases it can cause major physical and mental changes. The lowest level of testosterone for men is 300 ng/dL and the maximum is 1000-2000 ng/dL. How do you recognize the first indications of low T prior to being tested? What is the cause of low T?

The Sign1 - Sex Sign 1 - Sexual

As testosterone decline is common most men fear about the day when sexual desire and performance are affected. However, age is not necessarily the cause of low testosterone since the change takes time and low sex drive does not happen immediately. But there are three indications that your levels aren't enough:

Sex desire is reduced

Less spontaneous erections, like during sleep

Infertility

Do not confuse low testosterone with E.D. (erectile dysfunction). Testosterone is only playing a tiny part in this scenario. Testosterone therapy can help treat ED however it's not the reason.

Sign 2. Physical Changes

You know the reason why this hormone is referred to in the context of the hormone male, because it has male characteristics. It improves hair growth and muscle massand aids in the development of lean and strong muscles. If testosterone levels are low, physical changes may occur:

The body fat levels are an increase

Strength and mass decreases in muscles.

Fragile bones

Hairless body

Breast tissue tenderness or swelling

Fatigue is increasing

Hot flashes

The metabolism of cholesterol is affected.

Sign 3 - Sleep Disturbances

Although low testosterone can lead to low energylevels, it could cause sleep issues, such as shifts in sleeping patterns and, in some instances sleepiness. However testosterone therapy could cause sleep apnea which can disrupt sleeping pattern. The general changes to the body that result in sleep apnea may also be the reason for low T.

Sign 4 - Changes in Emotion

In addition to the physical changes, the levels of T can affect your emotions as well. The condition can cause depression as well as feelings of sadness. It can impact your overall well-being. There are instances where people suffer from problems with memory and concentration, and feel less self-confidence and motivation.

Because it is the hormone responsible for the regulation of emotions, depression can be often associated with men who have low levels of T. This could be because of fatigue, lower sexual motivation, or even irritation.

All-Over symptoms and signs of low T

Physical:

Energy loss, fatigue

The strength of muscles is reduced and mass

A rise in body fat

Back back pain

The bone density is reduced, which increases the likelihood of developing osteoporosis (more likely to suffer a bone fracture)

Heart attack risk

High cholesterol

Refractory period gets longer (increased interval between sexual encounters, and inability enjoy more frequent sexual encounters)

Sperm count can be reduced (infertility)

Gynecomastia (male breasts)

Mental:

Lower sexual drive, libido reduced

Brain fog, difficulty concentrating

Memory issues

Emotional:

Sadness, despair, hopelessness Depression

Motivation and ambition are reduced.

The disorder is known as Irritability (loss of patience, increased anger and anger)

Then Increase Your T

If you only follow the symptoms you notice or you have a test to determine the levels of testosterone (a basic blood sample) There is no quick fix to reach your goal of achieving testosterone. If you think you will get information about some magical supplement to your muscles then you're in the incorrect. There isn't one. The best choice is the way you live your life. It all comes down to what you do with your life. It's all about one thing: altering your lifestyle and diet in the long run. If you truly desire to achieve great T levels and stay in that state, it's crucial to follow the new way of life and be satisfied.

Diet

I was looking to avoid any other methods to boost testosterone since they will be done through intensive training. Testosterone levels increase when you are able to manage your stress levels and rest. This means that it is essential to live a healthy and balanced lifestyle to keep your levels under control.

Diet is crucial in the process of T production. The glands require specific minerals like zinc and magnesium to start production, and Leydig cells (in the testes) require cholesterol to produce testosterone. Foods such as broccoli, broccoli, and cauliflower boost T levels by eliminating estrogen from the body. There's no specific diet that you must follow, but you are able to make your own plan easily. You can only choose a handful of food items to adhere to:

Spinach is the best sources of magnesium are spinach. Not only can it enhance the growth of muscles, it is can also be essential to the reproductive function in both old, active and sedentary. Magnesium is recommended to be consumed at a rate of 22 mg for every pound. of body weight every day. If you are increasing your magnesium intake by increasing it, you'll boost your T levels. Also, make sure you eat lots of leafy greens , not just spinach. A cup of spinach (cooked) can provide you with about half of your daily intake It is also twice as much as you'll get from Kale.

Oysters are a great source of zinc, a mineral that can boost testosterone, while also increasing another vital hormone, called the growth factor (more about the growth factor in a bit). Training with zinc supplements have had amazing results within the first few weeks. Zinc supplements can boost testosterone levels as in boosting leg strength much more so than placebo.

Just six oysters (on the half shell) will provide you with 33 mg zinc. That is three times the amount (12mg per adult male).

Hot Sauce Make it hot! The more hot the pepper or pepper sauce, the higher testosterone you'll get. Studies have proven that the more hot you can consume, it indicates that your testosterone levels are high. It can also reduce belly fat and boost your size organs of sex. A lot of benefits can be found in simple hot sauce.

Garlic - There's the compound that is present in garlic that stimulates the hormone luteinizing. It's the one responsible for controlling testosterone production. The addition of garlic to a diet high in protein can boost T production. In reality, 500 mg of garlic or onion per 1 lb. each day will be sufficient to increase the T amounts by 30% within 20 days. Both garlic and onions have the exact chemical that produces the hormone that is responsible for the start of T production. It is important to note that fresh onions and garlic are rich in nutrients than powders.

Brazil Nuts The Brazil nuts are distinctive because they're rich in trace minerals like selenium. It is indeed an essential trace mineral however Brazil nuts provide the most potent source. It's been found that those who struggle with conception also have low levels of T and then low levels of selenium. Selenium levels increased for those who had their T levels under control and were able impregnate their partners.

Selenium is needed at a rate of 55 micrograms every day, and you will get approximately 90 mcg in one Brazil nuts.

So don't overeat! The maximum selenium intake is only 400 mg; and if exceeded, it could cause poisoning. So, don't go too nuts.

Broccoli The vegetable is cruciferous, and all varieties of it are high in the indoles, which can fight cancer and increase testosterone production indirectly through releasing and flushing out excess estrogen from the body. As we get older, estrogen levels increase and testosterone declines. Indoles vegetables will help ensure that they are in equilibrium. You can show that you know how to maintain your body through eating indoles Brussels sprouts and cabbage and broccoli.

Eggs - The boost in hormones that you receive from an egg comes resulted from the yolk. In actual. It has been established that vegetarians have 12% lower testosterone, and that an eating plan that is high in mono-saturated, cholesterol and saturated fats will increase testosterone. What is the reason for this? Simple cholesterol forms building blocks which are used to create T.

You can also enjoy an egg or two every week in whatever way you'd like. In order to have a balanced and healthy and balanced diet, eggs need to be included in your daily menu. Be mindful of quality over quantity.

Growth Hormone

The hormone is similar to testosterone as it has the same benefits. It reduces fat and boosts the size of muscles. It is not necessary to follow any special diet or adjustments in your lifestyle to increase the production of this hormone. All you have to focus on is exercising, eating healthy and get enough sleep. Within a short time all you need to do is make it work and you'll experience the boost you've been searching for.

When this hormone is in balance and you'll be more relaxed and of course you will be more energetic that will allow you to work out more. If everything is in sync you'll definitely lose weight and build the size of your muscles.

Growth hormones are made during sleep. And when you are sleeping less whatever what the cause (mostly stress) it can reduce production of this hormone.

What can you do to boost your growth hormone?

Sleep well every night (at minimum 8 hours)

Training for heavy weights

Niacin supplements, or including foods that are high in niacin into your diet (1-3gr daily)

Reduce the levels by insulin (limit carbs)

Insulin

The hormone produced by the pancreas is called insulin and its function is to transfer blood sugar or glucose to the cells that can later be burned to generate energy. Another important role of insulin is the movement of amino acids to promote anabolic activity. It's not a surprise that too much insulin can be an effective fat-building agent.

The pancreas plays a crucial function here since it releases digestion hormones as well as enzymes. It is located below the stomach and connects to the small intestinal tract.

How does insulin affect bodybuilding? It's simple, no matter if you're resistant or not. It is possible for a person to be more or less resistant to insulin , or in certain instances, sensitive to the hormone. According to the circumstances that cause it, it could become a medical issue and be an obstacle to building muscle and losing weight. The causes are:

Genetic predisposition

Stress and emotional stress

There isn't enough fat in the diet

Too much sugar intake

No exercising

Obesity

Insulin levels rise and stay elevated when carbohydrates are consumed in large quantities. Over time, cells adapt to carbs , and become resistant to the job. Insulin is a sugar transporter that carries sugar to cells to fuel. However, the excess that isn't being used to generate energy is converted into fat.

Because of not being able weight and build muscles, a variety of health problems may arise, including heart disease.

When you are doing intense weight lifting and conditioning the body requires more carbohydrates so that the intake of them regulates your energy. This means that more than the normal intake of carbohydrates is required both before and after exercise, approximately 50 grams prior to training and 60 grams following. Be sure to reduce your carb intake to ensure that there isn't any left to store fat.

Thyroid Hormone

The fourth most important hormone that is essential for fitness and health is thyroid hormone, that is responsible for controlling the body's temperature, and also controls our appetite, metabolism as well as mood and energy levels. If your thyroid hormone is not functioning properly it will cause you feeling tired due to the fact that your metabolism slows and the energy levels are less.

Like any other hormone stress can impact its performance. This is particularly true when you're constantly stressed. In this scenario, the immune system will not be able to function properly and your body will not be protected against viruses, for instance. As the thyroid begins to decrease metabolism, the body will begin to store calories in the form of fat. Therefore slower metabolism can lead to less energy levels.

If you're suffering with an inactive thyroid hormone The first sign you notice is fatigue. It's like feeling exhausted every day. (I had issues with this hormone, and it's not a good thing). There is no determination and drive to work out and adhere to a diet when they are tired and sleeping or napping can help the symptoms. Other symptoms include joint and muscle pain the skin becoming dry, itchy and dry. It can also be caused by slow growth of hair or evident shedding. The low levels of thyroid can lead to the retention of fluids that result in eye or face swelling, as well as puffiness of the feet, legs or hands. The lower the level of the hormone greater the production of cholesterol. Low or high concentration can lead to high blood pressure.

Chapter 2: Nutrition

We live in a culture where we are obsessed with the word calorie. On every other food item it is marked with a label proclaiming that there are no calories or very little. What is a calorie and why should we be concerned about each one that we take in? In reality, the calorie is crucial in our understanding of nutrition and diet. For a bodybuilder, there are three distinct categories to be concerned about. They are protein, fats and carbohydrates. In the following section, we'll go into greater detail about what each are, their reasons for being crucial, and the best way to incorporate them into your daily diet. In the meantime, here's an overview of the calories.

Human beings depend on calories to perform our daily tasks. Calories are the energy that the body requires to carry out daily tasks like regulating your heart rate, digesting your food and even breathing. Every food has a unique amount of calories . They comprise of carbohydrates as well as fats and proteins, also referred to as macronutrients. The variance for every person is based on the minimum amount of calories needed to live. The basal metabolic rate, also known as BMR can be altered based on the quantity of lean muscle mass a person has in their body. This can also impact the amount of calories you'll require to consume in a day. There are websites where you can input your age and height, sex, and weight to determine your BMR. Once you've done this then, you need to understand why macronutrients are essential for building muscle.

Protein

If there's one thing that you should know about bodybuilding and nutrition and bodybuilding, it's the fact that protein is a crucial element in the transformation of your body! Protein is why you can build muscles and not gain weight as women worry about. Lean muscle is the way women attain the toned, attractive appearance many people want. What exactly is it that protein has that can help build muscle?

Protein is composed of amino acids, which is the way your body produces muscle protein . It's also effective in aiding the development of muscle. When we work out that cause damage and tension to the muscles' fibers. In order to heal muscles, protein aids in the catabolism of muscles and heals it to ensure that you are better able to get stronger and more fit in a specific amount of time.

You know how proteins work but what amount should you consume? As we said earlier, some bodybuilders are identified as taking in excessive amounts of protein. Although this is an unflattering reality, it's vital. Protein intake too high can lead to constipation! This isn't a pleasant moment! Beware of excessive protein!

In general it is recommended that your protein intake consumed should be in line with one's body weight. If, for instance, you weigh 130 pounds, then you must aim to consume about 130g of protein. If you feel that this is an excessive amount of protein, keep in mind that it is possible to split it across many meals. Each meal, it is important to consider the protein, fats and carbohydrates you're taking into your body.

For proteins that are good for you There are many products that you can include into your diet to ensure that you are getting your daily protein intake. This includes items like eggs, beans, Greek yogurt, milk and soy, as well as nuts, and the quinoa. Each of these items are suitable for breakfast lunch, dinner, or both so that you can have your diet varied and never be bored!

Fats

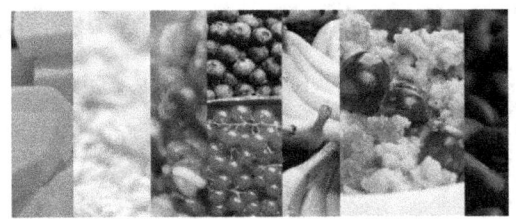

Like the calorie, the public seems to be obsessed with fats. Nowadays, many brands claim that they have no fat in their products. This is a popular mistake. However, the the content of fat is frequently misconstrued, and thus, get a negative reputation. Our bodies require fat in order to perform its functions! Certain, fat-free or reduced fat foods are a good choice when consumed in moderation, but so can healthy fats.

These healthy fats we're discussing are omega-6 and omega-3. This is the type of fat which help protect your organs and tissues as well as aid in the absorption of fat-soluble vitamins, aid in making you feel fuller after eating and help develop your brain! It's surprising that fat can be beneficial for your body. Keep in mind that all things are good when they are when it is done in moderate amounts!

Why was the federal government obsessed with weight gain in the first in the first As with everything, gaining weight is the result of having too many calories! This isn't due to excessive fat. It is simply calories that the body doesn't need and are therefore stored as fat to be used later. It's the trans-fats which you should avoid within your daily diet. Food manufacturers employ trans fats, such as hydrogenated oils in order to maintain their products on the shelves for longer. They are obviously not healthy for you. Instead, we recommend choosing healthy sources of fat, such as avocados, coconut oil grass-fed butter, nuts as well as olive oil. Remember to Keep these healthy fats in a small portions!

Carbohydrates

Carbs also have an unpopularity with fat. Contrary to what you've been told, carbs aren't the cause of problems! Much like the fats, you require them to help your body perform. You need a balance of carbohydrates, fats and protein in order to build the body you've always dreamed of.

If you cut any of them out, it will result in a disruption to the delicate chemistry that your body requires to become the best version of you!

Carbs are made of simple sugars with a single molecule and Double compound sugars. This is the process where three of the molecules are woven together that they form what is called a complete carb. Most of us they are more commonly found in the form of oatmeal as well as broccoli, potatoes and many other veggies. In terms of a diet, the majority of your carbohydrates should be from these complex carbohydrates. Complex carbs are why you are able to stay fuller for longer, and also get essential nutrients like vitamins, minerals, and fibers. In addition to these advantages, they ALSO aid in controlling the blood sugar level. It is recommended to look for foods like bananas, berries brown rice, brown rice, low-fat oatmeal, milk, vegetables (potatoes and broccoli, as well as spinach) as well as yogurt!

After you have a better understanding of the foods you should be eating It's almost as crucial to know the amount of food you're eating. The normal ratios of macronutrients ought to be around 40 percent carbs 30% protein, with 30 percent fat. While this is an average but it does not mean that it is suitable for all people. To determine the best ratio for you, you'll be required to identify your body kind. In the next chapter, we'll discuss female anatomy to help identify what type of woman you are.

One of the most effective methods to control the way you eat is being able to determine an appropriate amount. In America we are surrounded by excessive portions that are not enough for what's in our diets. Research has shown that those who have an abundance of food and justify their food and disregard when they are full. It is important to be aware of the food you put in your mouth and how much to your body.

Certain people are turning to calorie counting in order to keep the track of their portions and calories, however this isn't always the best choice. Research has proven that counting calories doesn't perform over the long term. In addition, calorie counting could sometimes be incorrect. With regards to serving sizes and the measurements it is often difficult to maintain consistency, and, in the end it's really the result of speculation. Instead, focus greater on macros and make certain that the food being served will keep your body fueled to time's end.

Chapter 3: Workout Plans

You require a lot of dedication to start your bodybuilding exercise. Contrary to popular opinion that you should exercise more often than experienced bodybuilders. The reason behind this is quite simple, experts are aware of the best ways to push their muscles, and consequently cause more harm to their bodies. This can take longer to recover from. in the beginning, your muscles may be sore, however, since you're not exercising your muscles to an extreme, you'll be able to return to action quicker.

In this case, damage isn't an unfun word! Don't worry about it the damage to muscles is a good thing in bodybuilding since it allows the body to recuperate by overcompensation (that increases the muscle's growth). This is precisely what bodybuilding is built on an ongoing cycle of repair, damage and growth that occurs on the course of a week.

When we refer to muscles are damaged, we're speaking of small tears on the muscles' fibres. Muscle soreness is also called DOMS (delayed soreness that develops at the time of onset) typically peak around 48 hours following exercise.

The exercise plan for this chapter was created to concentrate on just one area of the body every day on weekdays. The weekend is a time to rest the body, and allowing it to recover the strength and vitality. It is important to remember that this is only an outline. You can alter it as you need in order to achieve your goals for fitness.

Another thing you should remember to remember is to begin each workout with a warming up exercise. A warm-up session could be as easy as five minute in the gym. It prepares your body and mind for your workout.

After your workout, it is essential to cool down to stop the process from advancing and blood accumulating in your muscles. A cool-down will help to reduce the amount of adrenaline that builds up in your system throughout your workout. It could be a short exercise in stretching or a slow walk or running.

If you are a novice, be aware that you shouldn't overdo it in the beginning. Make sure that you use weights that aren't too heavy to hold, but make sure that the weights provide sufficient resistance. As you become stronger you will be able to gradually increase the weight you lift.

Day 1 - Upper Body:

Do the following exercises using two sets of 12 repetitions each:

* Dumbbell press

* Press your triceps in a reclining position

* Military press with standing barbell

* Situated dumbbell curl

* Preacher curls

* Dumbbell rows

* Side lateral raise

* Dumbbell shrugs

* Pec deck butterflys

* Lat pulls pulleys with pulley machine

* V-bar pushdowns

Day 2 - Abs and Lower Body:

Complete each of the following exercises in two sets of 12 repetitions each. For the crunches, you can complete as many of them as you'd like:

* Barbell squat

* Lunges

* One leg barbell squat

* Stiff leg barbell

* Calf press with standing

* Crunches

They are extremely helpful in sculpting your lower back. If you're exercising in a gym, then you might want to consider adding these machines exercises to your routine.

The leg presses are on a machine loaded with plates

* Hamstring curls sat on the floor

* Leg extension machine

* Ab machine

* Standing hamstring curls

Day 3 - Relax your body

Day 4 - Upper Body:

Once you've done the exercises for the first time, intensify the workout to three sessions of twelve reps each

* Chin ups

* Dumbbell presses on an inclined bench

* Hammer curls for dumbbells that are seated

* Standing in bicep curls

* Military press with standing barbell

* Upright barbell row

* Barbell tricep extension

* Front dumbbell raise

You can make use of the machines to complete the below exercises for Day 4:

* Cable rows that are sat.

* Cable crossovers fly.

* Cable rows that are upright

* Pushdowns of the Tricep Rope

Day 5 - Abs and Lower Body:

Reduce the exercise by two 12 repetitions with the exception of the crunches. You are free to perform the number of crunches you would like:

* Lunges

* Calf press with standing

* Barbell squat

* Standing calf raises

* Stiff leg barbell

* Crunches

The machine's exercises throughout the day, which include the following:

The leg presses are on a machine loaded with plates

* Kneeling hamstring curls\

* Hamstring curls that are seated

Weekend - Rest:

If the workout schedule of four days appears to be too strenuous it is possible to reduce it down to three-day or two-day plan. Remember that the results from less days may not be as apparent at the beginning. Beginning slowly can aid in building momentum for your next workout.

To assist you Here is a good example of a three-day exercise you can do:

Day 1 Back, Chest and Abs

Perform the following workout with three sets comprising 10-12 reps:

* Bent over barbell row

* Barbell bench press

* Barbell with stiff legs dead lift

* Incline dumbbell press

* Crunches

* Dumbbell flies

Day 2 Day 2 Legs and Shoulders

Repeat the exercise in three sets comprising 10-12 reps per set:

* Barbell squat

* Front dumbbell raise

* Calf raise seated

* Side lateral raise

* Lunges

* Upright barbell row

* Barbell squats

Day 3 Day 3 Biceps, Triceps, and Abs

Finally, you can conclude your week of fitness with the following exercises, in three sets of 10-12 reps per set:

* Barbell curl

* Pressing the triceps thigh muscles lying on your back.

* Incline dumbbell curl

* Front dumbbell raise

* Barbell tricep extension

* Hammer curls for dumbbells

* Crunches

After you've understood the exercise plan you'll be following, it's time be focused on your diet. A little more than an hour prior to the exercise, you will need to eat protein and carbohydrates to supply your body with the energy needed to complete the workout. If you eat the right foods, your body enters an anabolic state , which gives you the energy required to work your muscles efficiently.

While you exercise there is an increase in flow of blood to muscles which encourages growth of the muscles. If you consume the right amount of protein and carbohydrates prior to exercising the body gets the benefit of the increased blood flow and exercises the muscles accordingly.

Many people would prefer the rice bowl along and a protein shake prior to training, however you can pick any type of food you enjoy. Be sure to contain the essential nutrients for a fitness.

It is recommended to record your exercise routine. Write down the amount of reps and sets you do for every exercise (with the weight you're using) in a notebook or even on your smartphone. Gradually increase reps and set for every exercise throughout the exercise. Be sure to note the duration (or weeks number) along with the rest of the workout. This will help make sure you are aware of how long it takes to increase the number of reps and weights for the exercise.

Another tip to consider is to begin your first exercise with the smallest weight is possible. This will allow blood to start going through your muscle. After you've done the one set make more weights for the next set. If you find it difficult, you can increase the weight and do the third set.

Your aim should be to add weight until it becomes impossible to finish the sets i.e. until your muscles provide an resistance against the load.

Make sure to rest between two sets to allow your body to recuperate. The rest period should last under a minute since you don't want your muscles to become cold.

Additionally, it's a recommended to incorporate cardio exercises into your workout to increase the circulation of blood throughout the body. This could be as simple as an easy exercise like running on the treadmill. Cardio is not just beneficial to your body but also for the heart too. To avoid muscle breakdown , it is recommended to take a few easy BCA's prior to your workout.

Nutrition is one of the most essential factors that make up the success of a workout plan. This is the reason you have to be aware of what you must and shouldn't eat when developing muscles. In the next chapter, we will go over the specific eating practices you must follow to build muscle.

SWEET DREAMS

While sleeping is a crucial element of a workout routine however, it's overlooked a many times. If you are beginning an exercise program to build your body make sure you remember that rest is among the most beneficial tools to your development.

Your muscles grow and adapt especially at night. While you're in a suspended state of motion your body is actually building muscle , something you strive to achieve when you exercise.

Your body experience an intoxicating feeling when you don't sleep enough. Journal of Applied Sports Science discovered that staying awake for longer then 24 hours can be as good as having a blood alcohol level that is 0.096 (more than what is the legally-required limit for driving in many states) with regard to the physical effects.

Training when you is not sleeping well is not without its drawbacks and will not produce the desired results of exercise. In particular, the lack of coordination in your muscles will increase the risk of injuries. Like you wouldn't exercise after drinking a couple of glasses of alcohol and then head to the gym if are not sleeping the night prior. It is best to delay your training until the next day, after your body is getting enough rest.

What are the most effective things to do to ensure you get enough rest and adequate sleep? Here are some suggestions to assist you:

Do not exercise prior to getting ready to sleep. Sleeping is heavily affected by the temperature of your body. If it's lower, you begin to feel tired. If you sweat prior to bed it could take many hours to cool enough to help you go to sleep.

Eat a light meal prior to getting ready to go to go to bed. While some might do not agree with this idea but, sleeping with an empty stomach can distract our ability to sleep. But, ensure you are not eating something that is difficult to absorb.

You should sleep for at least 8 hours each evening. 8 hours of sleep will provide your body with the rest and recuperation it needs to perform efficiently throughout the day.

Make sure your bedroom is quiet and cool.

Avoid drinking too much drinks before bed Avoid caffeine-rich beverages like coffee or tea. In the first place, caffeine will cause you to stay awake. Additionally, you'll be forced to go to the bathroom more frequently, which could cause sleep disturbances.

Create a sleep routine prior to bed as well as establishing an established sleep routine. In this way, you will make sure that your body is ready to relax.

The body's protein synthesis is increased when you sleep This is the main reason behind the growth. The time you sleep provides the best chance the body has to repair and heal the damage it sustained throughout the daytime.

Many growing hormones can be released during an unwinding state. These hormones are crucial in boosting the size of your muscles. Growth hormones can also be released in the course of a workout, but the majority of them occur while you're asleep.

In addition to providing you with an increase in energy levels, sleeping can help your body recover and ultimately expand just as you'd like it to.

As we mentioned before If you truly want to build your body it is not a good idea to skip the supplements. But, they can be too complicated.

Chapter 4: Why it is important to build muscle

How Are Muscles?

The human body is comprised of diverse tissues, which include connective tissues, skin and organs, the nervous system and bone and body fluids. muscles. Muscles are soft tissue made from muscle cells which can expand and contract. Muscles create force and also the motion of our bodies.

How do muscles create force? Muscle cells make two filament proteins known as myosin and actin, which together form filaments of actomyosin. Actomyosin filaments are flexible, and they can be stretched and changed in size and shape. Their contraction can lead to the generation of force and the movement of muscles that results in the movements of organs that are linked to muscles.

There are three kinds of muscle: the cardiac muscles, smooth muscles , and the skeletal muscles.

The muscle of the Cardiac is located in the heart alone and is the sole source of heart's beating. The muscle in the heart is voluntary because it is not controlled by the brain.

Smooth muscles are found in the organ walls like stomach, esophagusand the urethra, blood vessels stomach, intestines and uterus and the bronchi. The smooth muscles can also be found on the skin, which controls the hair erection process. Similar to cardiac muscles smooth muscles, they aren't controlled by the brain.

Skeletal muscles are the largest kind of muscle that are responsible for generating human movements. They are primarily attached to bones in the skeleton they are the ones that control all actions we do consciously, such as eating, sitting, walking working, running, and working out. The majority of skeletal muscles are voluntary and managed by our brain.

When we focus on bodybuilding it is a way to build our muscles of the skeleton stronger and more powerful. It has numerous health benefits, which will be explained in the later portions in the text.

Muscle Building

The most important question in bodybuilding is how workouts and strength training result in muscle growth. When you perform exercises that require strength or weight your muscle fibers become broken and damaged. This causes the activation of a particular type of cell known as satellite cells which reside near muscle cells in the body. Satellite cells that are activated proliferate and then join with muscles fibers that are damaged to repair the damaged fibers stronger. Additionally, satellite cells trigger the synthesis of protein in muscles cells. In combination, these processes result in the muscles being enlarged and more robust than before the exercise. The result is increased muscle.

To maximize the effectiveness of a the bodybuilding exercise, it's essential to note that the growth of muscles does not occur while you are working out. Instead the growth and repair of muscles occurs following the workout, while you're taking a break. Therefore, eating a balanced diet and getting a proper rest are essential to bodybuilding.

A few bodybuilders engage in excessive intense workouts without adequate rest, which can cause muscle soreness that is over a safe and healthy level. After workouts, they experience it difficult to complete any routine physical activity. This is due to the fact that the excessive exercises have surpassed the body's capacity to heal the injured muscles. This type of overtraining could cause injuries, and can slow the process of building muscle. Therefore, you must determine your body's capabilities of repair to muscles and make sure you don't overload your body.

Muscle Growth Hormones

You've probably heard about growth hormones for muscles. They're signaling molecules that regulate satellite cells as well as muscle cells throughout the body. The muscle satellite cells can be stimulated with growth hormones like Hepatocyte Growth Factor (HGF) and Fibroblast Growth Factor (FGF). The pituitary gland is the master gland that regulates the release of growth hormones.

Hepatocyte Growth Factor regulates satellite cell functions through causing satellite cells to move to muscles that are damaged to repair them.

It is believed that the Fibroblast Growth Factor is involved in muscle repair through stimulating the formation of blood vessels that are new, which means that more minerals nutrients proteins, oxygen and minerals are transported to muscles for growth and repair.

The Testosterone hormone and the Muscle growth

Testosterone is a hormone steroid which is produced through the testicles and the ovaries in women and men and women, respectively. Testosterone helps to build muscle as well as muscle strength, and increases strength and bone mass. Because testosterone levels in males are higher than those of women males generally have bigger muscles than women.

The secretion of these hormones through regular exercise as well as healthy eating and sleeping routines. If your body isn't able to produce sufficient growth hormones, you may want to consider taking supplements for growth hormones that boost the production of growth hormones throughout the body. However, the growth hormone supplements could cause serious adverse consequences and are only recommended and monitored by a skilled doctor.

What are the Benefits of Muscle Building

Everyone wants to be healthy and strong. A healthy and strong body is the basis for our overall health our life and even our professional career. Here are a few benefits of building muscle mass:

Strong muscles allow us to get the most enjoyment from exercise, sports, and other physical activities.

* Bodybuilding exercises can reduce cholesterol levels and lower the chance of developing heart disease, strokes or diabetes. It can also help prevent certain types of cancer.

Strong muscles strengthen our joints , and can protect us from fractures or injuries as we get older. Training to build muscles increases bone density, that are essential for preventing osteoporosis, a bone disease.

A well-toned body makes our appearance attractive and increases confidence in yourself.

* Bodybuilding can help us shed weight, no matter our age or gender.

Weight Loss Benefits

Lean and strong muscles aid us to burn more calories than fat tissues. Since it takes more energy to keep the mass of a pound of muscle than it does a pounds of fat, people that build up muscle will burn more calories than those with lesser muscle. Even when they are not exercising is the case, more calories need to be burned to sustain an athletic body as opposed to a body that has poor muscular tone and excessive fat.

If you exercise hard your muscles will be injured. In order to repair and grow, these muscles require energy that is partly generated by the fat burning process within the body. Muscle development also increases your metabolism, resulting in greater fat and calorie burning.

Chapter 5: The Basic Training Principles

Specificity: If your goal is to be a part of the Miss Olympia stage you are going to train a different way than a home wife who's focusing on strengthening your middle post her third baby. This is the concept behind specificity. For a specific outcome, you need an exact training plan. Therefore, you are using the weights to help to accomplish your goals. A good example of the principle of specificity can be basketball players. The principle states that the exercises he picks are similar to the ones he performs when on court. For the legs, he could select squats, or opt for leg extensions. Squats are more like the jump movements that are that are required for basketball, while leg extensions are an exercise that is isolated. Basketball players will choose to perform squats.

(2) Overload The overload principle implies that you have to always be lifting more weight doing more repetitions or reducing your interval rest time compared to your last exercise.

(3) Progressive Resistance: The concept of progressive resistance dates back in time to Milo of Croton who was a 6th century BCE wrestler. The legend says that as a young boy, Milo started carrying a baby calf each day when it was growing to maturity. The calf gained weight every day, however, since the size of the increase was so tiny, Milo didn't notice them. When the bull was at mature, Milo was able to transport it around the family farm. Weight trainers have drawn the inspiration of Milo since. When you increase the weight by tiny increments every workout it will allow you to drastically increase your strength that will

increase your fitness and increase the results of your fat loss.

(4) The intensity: The intensity refers to the amount of effort you devote to your workouts. If you're working at a high level of intensity, then the last 2 or 3 reps of each set must be difficult to complete. If you've finished the set and think you can do another set of 2 or 3 reps, you're not exercising at the right level of intensities. It is necessary to add weight, add reps or lower the rest in between sets.

(5) Rep Range: A rep's range refers to the amount of times that you can perform a specific exercise. To maximize the benefits of your training, you must to make sure you're performing the right number of repetitions for your particular goal in training. The standard rep range is as follows 4-7 reps for strength, 8-12 reps to

build muscles 13-20 reps for endurance and fat loss

(6) Volume The volume refers to the amount of reps and sets required for optimal performance. This subject is the subject that has been the subject of debate with those who advocate for extremely small volume exercise (one set for each exercise) and citing research studies to back their claims with the same passion as those who believe in large-volume training (20 sets for each section of body). The best approach is between the two. 3-4 sets per work set seems to be the ideal number.

(7) Rest (7) Rest between sets is vital. It can be as small (30 minutes) to extremely long (3 minutes or more). You'll need time to recuperate from the previous set so that you can complete an out effort for the next set. If you are resting too long the

intensity will remain at the same degree. You must build up each set before moving onto the next. This is why you should be resting for six seconds between sets.

(8) Tempo The word "tempo" is used to describe the speed at that you complete your repetitions. Each rep is made up of two distinct components, those of the lift (concentric) in addition to the downwards (eccentric). In the concentric portion of the lifting the muscle is shortening or contracting. It is lengthened during the eccentric part of the exercise. It is essential to utilize a steady tempo that lets you restrict the muscle that is working and prevent momentum from the lifting. The ideal training pace is two seconds to complete the concentric portion of the move and then 4 seconds for the eccentric portion. The eccentric portion of the exercise actually strengthens muscles more than the concentric portion. Slower

movements resist gravity and intensifies the exercise.

(9) Modification: Continually altering your training program can prevent your body from getting used to the load being put on it. This can help keep from reaching plateaus in training as well as keeps the body thinking and reacting. It also stops boredom from training and lets you exercise your body from different perspectives. The best way to keep your schedule fresh is to modify it each six-week period.

(10) Recuperation (10) Recuperation: When you exercise you put pressure on your body. The energy reserves are exhausted, muscle tissue is damaged and your body is placed in a state of fatigue. After the workout, it is that the recovery and rebuilding process takes place. This is

why you should take an interval of 48 hours between workouts.

Chapter 6: Training and Exercise Equipment

The athletes are well-aware of the notions that reps (repetitions) as well as sets (cycles of repetitions). Each one has its own merits and use.

Reps go through three phases:

The Concentric Phase This is the phase of muscle shrinking which is part of the lifting that you perform when you lift the dumbbell or throw the shotput. It is suggested to breathe out during your Concentric Phase.

Eccentric Phase: This is the phase that lengthens muscles. It's portion of a workout that allows you to reduce the weight and control the speed. Inhale when you are in this phase too. Many athletes overlook this stage, even though it is the time when the muscles are working to lift heavier loads. The more weight you can do, the better improve.

Isometric Phase: this stage in which the body is in tension but is not lengthening or shorterening; it's contracting but maintaining its length. Keep your breathing steady in this stage. One example of this is when you press against any object that is immovable, such as the wall of an area. The muscles in your body are working however your arms aren't moving and neither does the wall. The main drawback of this phase can be that your muscles during this stage aren't moving through the entire movement. The only advantage that can be realized is in how much range you demonstrate during your exercise.

"Volume" is the term used to describe how much work performed per rep. One method to determine volume is to measure the amount of work being performed by each muscle group or body part per week/workout; the amount per exercise as well as per workout week. If you want to build muscle reps, you should set your reps to 6-12 and sets 3 to 6. Lower than 6 will help build strength and power , but little bulk. Reps greater than twelve will lead to greater endurance, and smaller. The benefit of keeping track of the amount of weight is that if you take on too much, you run the risk of being detrimental to your body's ability heal itself and recover from injury. It reduces the likelihood of achieving the results you desire.

Keep your sets and reps within the guidelines above. Here's how that balance is attained (a fitness trainer, or a physical therapist could be of assistance here):

Try to work out every major upper body muscle section. When you think of the fact that there are over 665 skeletal muscles that are found in your body it is easy to understand why they are separated into groups. A few of them can be classified as "Major" muscles groups. Major muscles are the most powerful of all muscle groups. They are the ones that influence all of our movements. They are assisted by synergists, smaller muscles. The synergist muscle types include brachialis Serratus, rhomboidsand intercostals, erector Spinae and many others. As powerful and large as these muscles are, they require assistance to function. Find the right exercise for each, taking into account your objectives, the level of training, your personal abilities and limitations, as well as the limits and capabilities for the exercises. While you are working through these exercises, you'll be working out a variety of muscles that are smaller.

Balance: This fundamental concept is often forgotten when someone is preparing their training program. The world is full of different things happening constantly in our lives that we often forget what we're trying accomplish. Balance is essential for maximum performance. If you are able to adjust your training program so that it is compatible with your other activities you'll be in balance.

Here are some important things to keep in mind: sometimes life can stop us from doing the things we'd like to accomplish. Events happen that aren't within our control. The news can be good or negative, but in any case it will impact our performance. If you've made training a priority, make the date on your schedule. So you'll have less chance to forget to note things in the wrong location. If it happens again, don't get upset. This is the way life works.

The importance of competition is that it gives you the chance to start your training against the most rigorous standards. It is the perfect opportunity to display all of your hard work in front of an audience of supporters who will be cheering for you. The pressure of competition is for the body and mind throughout the entire process. However, bodybuilding can help athletes become stronger, improve their endurance and improve their health throughout. There are sacrifices to be made such as time away from home activities, hobbies, or even obligations. Bodybuilding isn't just a hobby It's a lifestyle that advanced athletes take on.

When bodybuilders consider competition, envision being in a contest. They aren't meant for everyone. They're designed to let you know the qualities you have. To stand up to these obstacles, you must have an enlightened and well-conditioned mind. The event will be filled with numerous obstacles, so the better prepared you are, the more successful you will be.

Choose wisely when selecting your contests. They can be fun however, you'll be smart to look them over to figure out which are your major events for the year. Which is the most beneficial for you. Which one is most appealing to you.

When you compete, there are distractions. It is not wise to suggest athletes not talk or visit when they are in the gym However, if you're trying seeking to be balanced it is essential to keep distractions to the minimal amount. Pick a signal to signal that you're prepared to begin your workout: tap your foot, whistle, or any other signal that can signal your intentions.

A positive attitude towards your work is crucial. This will keep your focus on the task instead of quitting or slowing down. Positive results can help you stay in concentration. Be aware that better results are because of a balanced approach to exercising and resting. You are the only one who can determine when it's the right time to end your workout, or put your feet down and give your muscles time to recuperate and rest. Try your best and don't go overboard.

It is essential to have both long-term and short-term goals that keep you on track and on the right track. If you're training for the marathon, your goals for training will differ from goals of those who are looking to shed weight. The first step is to focus on strength training over the next 7 to 9 weeks. Then, you'll need to lift exercises three times a week.

To improve your flexibility and mobility You can try yoga. Running can reduce the mobility of some joints since it doesn't allow ankles or hips to exercise their entire range of movement. If you don't have the time to go to an yoga class, you can try to squeeze into your schedule a couple of exercises designed specifically for athletes. A few yoga poses that you can incorporate into your fitness routine are the dog that is facing downwards the lunge with a high angle, the twisted lunge, dolphin and the Pigeon. Yoga can help increase your strength as well as increase your muscle mass. If your other activities, sports like bicycling, running, or swimming have left you with weak muscles, yoga may help you make up for the lack here. The stability of your core will increase while the risk of injury due to overuse is minimized. All in all, you'll end with more stable and efficient strength. There is nothing better than increasing your results faster from your training

Workouts that rely on the body alone include lunges, pushups etc.

There are a variety of machines available to select from:

The treadmill can be very effective in burning calories, with an average of 100 miles per hour. Many have adjustable settings to fit your needs, and you can set the incline for instance, very soft. But, anyone with joint pain or is overweight might consider walking a bit unpractical. When your foot touches it's feet, its force is 3.7 times the weight of your body. If, after you have adjusted the treadmill to your preference, you feel there's still pain after the workout, you should consider an alternative machine. There might be balance issues associated with using the treadmill too particularly for beginners and those that haven't exercised recently.

Machines for rowing: These offer a full exercise, especially in the cardio zone. The rowing machines test you to coordinate: they make you work your abs in order to build the upper part of your body. When you push your body back you shoulders, rear, and arms have to work. The harder you work and the more you push them, the stronger they become. Also, you can expect to experience a greater heart's strength as well as an increase in your body's capacity to burn calories effectively.

Elliptical machines and stairs steppers: These devices are an effective alternatives to treadmills. They are less stressful on joints, and as they require you to stand up when using these machines, you are using lots of muscles and burn a lot of calories.

Stair steppers are more effective instead of running down and up the bleachers. As with all other machines the stair steps are detrimental to your posture. Many beginners believe it's cool, even at their very first attempt, to crank the machine to the highest setting while ignoring their posture. This isn't very cool. In the end, they're grasping their rails, or leaning over, transferring the weight of their legs onto their arms or onto the machine, leading to less calories being burning.

To solve this issue To solve this issue, place your hands against the bars or side rails with no grip. Turn down the speed until are confident that you will maintain the speed of your machine. Gradually increase the speed, but slowly. Make sure you keep your entire pedal in place to strengthen your back and thighs Avoid over-taxing the muscles in your calf.

The stationary bike: experts believe that the stationary bike is a great exercise that is the least impacts on joints. Anyone suffering from knee pain might find these bikes to be easy to ride, since the impact on joints is lesser. Be sure that the bike has been fitted for your physique by an skilled person. A good fit is crucial. Be sure to sit in the bicycle with the sole of both your legs on the pedals and your knees bent slightly. Avoid, using this posture the knees being allowed to bend too much, as this could cause too much pressure to your knee, causing pain.

If the impact of impact is a concern for you, skip the treadmill and go for cycling. Do not use rowing machines at this point. Do not overdo it in the beginning; for those who are just starting out as much muscle work and the more you work, the faster you'll overwork yourself and also consume fewer calories.

Chapter 7: Two Step Process

Ripping is a two step procedure.

1. Build

2. Chisel

Your body functions like an object, and you're creating an image of a statue. The first step is to create the general shape, and after that you chisel and cut down the statue to reveal the finer details. To get rid of it, you'll have to be an artist. You are the body sculpture you're making and you're the one who's sculpting it and making it.

If you're a sculptor who is creating the statue, adding more over a built is a mistake. Why would you continue to build instead of cutting down the statue to reveal the finer details? Then , after chiseling for details, you build and again. Then, after you have built more, you chisel further. Continue this process until your statue is tall enough and has all the necessary details.

That's how you make the statue, and this is the way you're damaged. Building more will eat more. Chiseling means eating less. This is known as cutting and bulking in bodybuilding terms. I'm not a fan of those words however. We're not bodybuilding , we're statue-sculptors who sculpt our bodies.

It's an easy process, but the majority of people fail in this area. I see large, fat individuals working out often. They're lifting heavyand getting stronger, but they're still looking like the shite of their lives. They're building constantly and never ever chiseling. There's no detail in their statue since it's made of huge blocks of bronze that require chiseling down to expose any form of detail.

If you're carrying too many large chunks of bronze, you're probably not building muscle effectively. The more fat you've got, the more difficult it will be to build muscles. Efficiency is the speed at which building muscle. The body can build muscle the most efficiently about 10-13 percent body fat. Achieving a body fat percentage of 20% and thinking you're getting larger is what makes me giggle. There's no way to gain muscles; the majority of the fat you're losing is.

Once you've figured out what to avoid and what not to do, I'll tell you how to proceed. It is best to begin building your body when you're with a slim body fat percentage, ideally 8-12 percent body fat. It is recommended to build for approximately 3 months before you work on it for two months. This is how I've been the most effective in my shaping. You'll look ripped and fantastic all year round. The majority of people look great when they cut their hair for the summer time. It's a good idea to look nice throughout the year.

When you begin building, this is what you'll accomplish; I refer to it as an incremental build. It's a gradual increase in the amount you eat each week during the first month of building. In week 1, you'll eat less than when you were making chisel. Week 2 you'll consume less than week 1. Week 3 will be less than week 2. Week 4 will be slightly more than week 3. You're now eating more than you did just a month ago, when you were working. In the last 2 months of your build, eat what you're eating after four weeks of growing.

In the initial month of building, you're creating your metabolism and body to build. Once you've made it through the one month building phase, your body will be ready for packing the muscle thanks to what you're eating. That's the reason you need to take 3 months to build and two months of chiseling. initial month to build is designed to increase your metabolism and get your body in shape to build muscles.

Simple, simple. When you're working on your building, eat more. when you're chiseling , eat less. The simplicity of your approach will allow you to achieve your goals. The majority of people confuse this with supplements, diets, nutritional plans and the like.

Chiseling and construction are suitable when you have the material to build statues. If, for instance, you're just beginning to work out, then you'll never be construction or chiseling. Instead, you'll be collecting bronze to make your sculpture and get the tools necessary to make it. Your body is transforming into an image of a statue. It's building muscle while burning fat while doing it. It's amazing that when you first begin working out , you'll get the highest and fastest results. The first year of exercising will produce the best results. After the first year's results do not appear, so that's why you build and grinding.

The human body was not created to have a huge, muscular muscles on it. It's against the human tendency to build inhuman muscles; to make an erect statue from our bodies. This is where chiseling and building is involved. Human bodies were designed to be muscular and lean but it was not designed to be ripped and large however.

It's not a problem because we're sculptors who mold our bodies into statues.

Chapter 8: Benefits of Carbohydrates for Bodybuilding

Carbohydrates are vital for bodybuilders, as they give them the energy needed to power their workouts and to ensure their muscles are filled with glycogen (which helps to give their muscle's full, round appearance) and also to stop the degeneration of the muscle tissue.

Carbohydrates are divided in two groups that are complex and simple carbohydrates.

Complex carbohydrates differ from simple carbohydrates due to the fact that they are made up of numerous bonding between carbohydrates (polysaccharides). Simple carbohydrates however are either single compounds (monosaccharides) or contain only the one bond that connects two compounds (di-saccharides).

The most commonly used form of carbohydrate bodybuilders prefer to consume is rice. While it's not a terrible source of carbohydrates, there are likely better alternatives from a health and nutrition viewpoint.

Rice isn't the most nutritious source of carbs for bodybuilders

There are a variety of reasons rice may not be the ideal carbohydrate for bodybuilders.

A concentrated source of carbohydrates

It is, first of all, an extremely high-concentration source of carbohydrates, which is why it triggers an important insulin response in the body. Although this is a good thing after exercising since it boosts anabolism within the body, it's not the best when it comes to other occasions, simply because elevated levels of insulin can also trigger the storage of fat.

Low in fiber

The type of rice most often consumed is white rice. Because white rice grains have been stripped of their husks by processing, the fiber content has been significantly decreased. Fibre is known for its various benefits for health, and decreasing its amount means the nutrition value of rice also gets diminished.

High Glycaemic Index

Fiber, especially insoluble fibres, can slow down carbohydrate absorption. So, the removal of most of the fibre from rice results in it having a higher the glycemic index (GI). Although this is not an issue if rice is eaten as part of the "complete meal" (with an oil and protein source) since the fat, protein and perhaps fibre from other ingredients included in the meal will lower the GI level of the rice.

A low amount of phytonutrients.

While rice contains some phytonutrients (nutrients taken from plants) but it tends to be lower than other food items. The majority of phytonutrients are found in fruits and vegetables that are rich and vibrant in colour.

The most effective carbs for bodybuilders should meet the following requirements:

High in Fibre

Moderate Carbohydrate Content

Low to Moderate Glycaemic Indice (GI)

The product is high in phytonutrients (nutrients that come from plants)

In this chapter, we'll discuss each of these points in greater specific detail.

High in Fibre

Fibre provides a variety of health advantages, making it an integral component of the diet of all. Here are some of the advantages they provide:

Absorbs carbohydrates slower

Lowers cholesterol levels.

Reduces time to transit through the gastro-intestinal tract (food moves through the digestive tract more quickly). This decreases the risk of colon cancer.

Offers food to the 'good bacteria that live in the gut.

The binding of toxic chemicals within the stomach

It reduces hunger

Certain foods rich in complex carbohydrates also high in fiber include legumes (beans peas, lentils) as well as fruits vegetables, oats, barley, chia, rye and corn.

Moderate Carbohydrate Content

The ideal carbohydrates for bodybuilders must have a moderate amount carbohydrates. The carbohydrate-rich food is thought to have a moderate amount of carbohydrates if most of it is made up of water and fibre.

This means it's possible to consume more quantity of food and be fuller more quickly. This also means that it will be more manageable to regulate calories as well as blood sugar levels and the insulin response and help people remain in top shape while building muscles.

The carbohydrates that meet this requirement are legumes, some fruits and the majority of vegetables.

Low to Moderate Glycaemic Indice (GI)

Carbohydrates that have a moderate to low GI are ideal for bodybuilders to eat. Although GI isn't a factor when a carbohydrate source is consumed as part of a "complete meal', it's important to focus on moderate to low GI complex carbohydrates in your diet.

For the record, the most nutritious carbohydrates include legumes, a few fruits, and a majority of vegetables.

The product is high in phytonutrients (nutrients taken from plants)

There are many kinds of phytonutrients found in plants, which nutritional science is only beginning to uncover. They are most abundant in foods with vivid, vivid hues.

The phytonutrients offer a variety of health benefits. They are especially beneficial in preventing illnesses that are prevalent in our modern society.

Additionally, because various carbohydrate sources come in distinct colours, they also contain various phytonutrients. This is why it's ideal to consume a range of carbohydrates in all your meals, to ensure that you provide your body with an array of phytonutrients.

A good source of carbohydrates for building muscle

Here are some carbohydrates (both simple and complex carbs) which are worth to include in your daily diet: strawberries, blueberries apple, bananas sweet potato, pumpkin, corn, peasand eggs, plant squash, zucchini English tomatoes, spinach cucumbers, etc.

A majority of these carbohydrate sources are covered on Chapter 10. Macronutrient Information Table in Chapter 10. The most effective sources of carbs for bodybuilding are typically those that are classified as low or medium-density carbohydrates.

As you will observe, there are better carbs-rich foods for bodybuilders to eat rather than the standard, old rice! When you incorporate these carbs into your diet on a daily basis, you're more likely to be easier to adhere to your diet in the for the long haul, enjoy your meals, remain in good form, and most of all, keep your optimal health!

The only occasion to experience high levels of insulin

It is essential to maintain a low level of insulin most of the time to ensure that the body can get access to the stored body fat as fuel.

But, insulin is among the body's top anabolic hormones. That means that it is able to dramatically boost the growth of muscles! So, having a high levels of insulin at certain times can be beneficial.

The ideal time to get an increase in the level of insulin within your bloodstream would be following exercise. The reason it's beneficial since insulin promotes the absorption of nutrients into your muscle cells . This can have a huge cell-volumising impact. Additionally, you are more likely to store those nutrients in fat because you are in a state of depletion.

Your body is exhausted after exercise is the reason it's fine to eat more carbs at the beginning of the day when you eat breakfast. Because your body has been without food for several hours, it's most likely to be a bit depleted. This is why it's okay to consume a little more carbs for breakfast but without adding weight.

Chapter 9: Andarine S4

Andarine S4 is another type of selective androgen receptor modulators (SARMS). Andarine S4 belongs to research chemical class. It binds to androgen receptor in the same way as regular androgens. However, the difference is that selective anabolic activity is produced by SARMS.

What are the uses for Andarine S4 is used for?

The advantage of Andarine S4 use in comparison to testosterone and anabolic steroids is there is no have to worry about muscles that aren't skeletal and undergo androgen actions. Andarine S4 can also be utilized to treat various medical illnesses. It is actually used to address:

*Muscle weakening

*Benign Prostatic Hypertrophy

*Osteoporosis

Andarine S4 is an oral product that assists in the development the lean muscle mass. It may also assist in increasing the quantity of muscle mass that is lean. A lot of people utilize it to increase their abilities and create the body they really want.

The method of use is dependent on the outcomes the user seeks. Losing body Fat (cutting) can be described as the method in which Andarine S4 use is the most efficient. The most popular steroids used in cutting include Winstrol, and Anavar. These steroids do not provide huge gains in the size of your muscles. However they are helpful in making your body leaner. Selective androgen receptor modulators possess similar properties to steroids. However, they are able to provide similar results, but without the negative consequences that involve the retention of water.

Dosage

The standard dosage to cut is 50mg over a 6 - 8 weeks. The regimen should consist of taking the drug every day for five days, then taking two days off over the time period. The dose taken every day during the duration of the cycle could cause changes in vision.

How Andarine S4 Functions

The advantages of Selective androgen Receptor Modulators are potential for bodybuilders or athletes and the benefits they can bring to certain medical diseases. They function by connecting to the receptor for androgen. This results in an increase in muscle mass. As the binding and activation process takes place it is also a source of protein created, which permits the muscle to develop. Andarine S4 could result in the growth of muscles that is like the results one can achieve with different types from anabolic steroids. In contrast, SARMS don't give adverse reactions similar to those on the prostate or other organs of sexual reproduction.

The benefits of Andarine S4

There are many advantages of Andarine S4 over the use of other anabolic steroids. These include:

There is no need for a pre-cycle

*Less expensive

*There is no evidence of estrogen-related adverse consequences

There is no risk to the liver.

Complete sense of well-being

*No water retention

*Reports

Many studies have been done using Andarine S4. Consuming 3 mg of Andarine S4 daily can aid in the restoration of skeletal muscle and resulting in results on laboratory rats. The study, which lasted 120 days using Andarine S4 as well as DHT in rodents confirms that bone strength and mass at higher levels were observed through Andarine S4 than DHT.

Research has proven that the use of Andarine S4 can result in weight loss and build lean muscle mass. These goals could also be accomplished in less time than if one would be using steroids. Although Andarine S4 is consumed orally and is not a risk for the liver, which is why it's a good thing to consider. It also doesn't cause problems due to excessive estrogen within the body.

Potentially harmful side effects of Andarine S4

There are a few possible adverse effects you should be aware of when you decide to take Andarine S4. Changes in vision is the most well-known consequence associated with Andarine S4. It is likely to occur in the event that Andarine S4 consumes in greater dosage. If this happens, lower the amount you take. The vision problems could result in difficulties in seeing at night or having a yellow hue. Vision changes cease following Andarine S4 has been eliminated present in the body.

Nutrobal (MK-677)

Nutrobal or MK-677 can be taken orally and is also an endocrine. Another term for the chemical substance that stimulates growth hormone is called secretagogue. Also, it is possible to connect it with several proteins like GHRP-6, or Ipamorelin. The Nutrobal however does not require injections and does not have any adverse side effects as well. It was originally developed to combat conditions like muscular weakness, obesity and osteoporosis. Its primary function employed for was treating hip issues among the elderly and you'll be aware that there's been a myriad of studies that prove the safety of this product to consume.

How MK-677 Functions

If you examine the strength of the pulse that growth hormone produces, you'll notice that it operates in four different ways. You can increase your GHRH that is the hormone for growth discharge hormone, and notice the increase in the GHRH. Additionally there is a decrease of the somatostatin discharge as well as the somatostatin receptor displaying as well. Nutrobal functions by releasing all four of these vital components . When you've taken it in, it increases the dosage prescribed. There are numerous reports about this type of drug and the studies were mostly based using the catabolic condition. If you are taking a daily dose of 25mg per day and you're on diet that has nitrogen wasting , then you'll experience a higher level of IGF-1. In addition the specific effects of nitrogen wasting were completely reversed. This indicates that it could be used to aid in the treatment of those suffering from muscle weakness, so there's a lot of benefits when looking the issue from this perspective. When tests were conducted on overweight and GHS and GHS, the results showed that there was an obvious increase in the muscle mass, and visceral adipose tissues did not seem to be affected. If you take Nutrobal for about 2 weeks, you'll notice a rise in basal metabolic rate and be aware that your mass of your body is boosted as well. There are other reports that have been conducted and it is clear that Nutrobal is a viable option to treat osteoporosis as well as bone mineral issues. It improves bone density, as well as aiding with any healing time.

The benefits of MK-677

There are many benefits to Nutrobal users. They can reap the benefits of improved skin as well as a boost in energy levels, and nitrogen retention as well. Additionally, you will discover that if you eat Nutrobal that you have an increased level of energy and a high level of health. In addition, your immune system will also be enhanced to realize that the benefits remain for a long time and are very effective as well. In fact research has shown that Nutrobal is a great supplement for a myriad of reasons including building muscle mass , cutting, and other. It isn't a threat to the number of additional hormones that are produced by HGH which makes it possible to consume it with an injection of HGH If you want. If you take Nutrobal You will be able to see that you can reap certain advantages without the need for intense HGH injections, and it's definitely not as difficult for you to enjoy all the benefits without worry or stress.

Some other benefits include muscle mass growth weight reduction, tightening loose skin increased bone mass, faster healing time and many other benefits. If you're interested in knowing the quantity of Nutrobal you should consume The recommended dose ranges from 5mg and 25mg per day. The dosage will depend on the results you would like to see.

Affects on MK-677's Side Effects

A few of the negative reactions that are typically associated with Nutrobal are fatigue as well as numb hands. increasing desire to eat. If you are taking Nutrobal over a long duration, then you'll notice you Cortisol levels will not rise, which is a huge issue when it's something you are concerned about. There are some evidence that show an initial increase in prolactin for some people after they started taking Nutrobal. However it is only evident for those who are sensitive to the prolactin-related effects. If this is the case for you, then you might consider taking an HCGenerate E to prevent any further complications. In what way can you tell whether you're prone to prolactin sensitivity? Examine your previous intakes. If you suffer from gynecomastia after the use of trenbolone, there is the possibility that you are sensitive to prolactin, so this is something you should be thinking about. Nutrobal however is a great way to increase your immunity, so it's worth talking to your physician if you are interested in learning more about what this medication can be able to do for you.

Chapter 10: What is the The Best Diet for Muscles Building?

1. Devour breakfast. The energy boost starts in the beginning of the day and will be less hungry throughout the day. This also sets the tone and you'll tend to eat more healthily if your day starts with a healthy and nutritious breakfast.

Your best bet for quality eggs: Omelets, smoothies and cottage cheese. Find a method to create the habit of eating breakfast.

2. Consume 3 times a day. The most convenient method: breakfast and lunch, dinner after exercise, pre mattress, and snacks in between. Advantages:

A lesser amount of starvation. By eating smaller meals, vs. eating a handful of large meals can decrease the size of your stomach. You'll feel fuller faster while your waist will slim.

There are fewer cravings. In fact, not eating for long intervals usually results in overeating the next meal, or ending on the sweet gadget.

Consume at regular times every day and your body will become hungry in those specific times. Example: 7am, 10am, 1pm, 4pm, 6pm, 7pm & 10pm.

3. Eat protein every day. Protein is essential to build and maintain muscles. Proteins can also aid in fat loss because they possess the greatest thermal impact. Proteins also help in satiating: they keep you fuller longer than carbohydrates.

How much protein should you take in each day? At a minimum, 1g of protein equivalent to the pound of body weight.

It's 200g a day if that you are 200 pounds. The most effective way to reach that amount would be to eat an entire protein source with every meal.

A few are:

Beef. Pork, red meat lamb, deer, buffalo, and more.

Rooster. Hen duck, turkey, and many more.

Fish. Tuna, salmon, sardines, mackerel, etc.

Eggs. Don't believe cholesterol myths. Take the yolk.

Dairy. Cheese, milk Quark cheese or cottage cheese yogurt, and so on.

Whey. Not as essential, but a great source to make clean exercise shakes

4. Enjoy a healthy diet of fruits and vegetables at every meal. The majority of them are low-calorie, meaning you can eat your stomach full without adding fat or weight. The greens and fruits are rich in nutrients, minerals and antioxidants as well as fiber, which aids in digestion.

Some of my most-loved fruits and vegetables include such as berries, apples and pineapples, as well as bananas, oranges tomatoes, broccoli beans, pumpkin, cauliflower, Brussels sprouts, bok chop, roman lettuce, chicory, peas and peas.

5. Consume carbs after a workout in the simplest way. Although you need carbs to provide power, many individuals consume much more that they actually need. Reduce your carb intake to complete your workout at the highest level.

Take fruits and veggies along alongside all your meals. They are low in carbs when as compared to whole grain. Exception: corn, carrots, raisins.

Other carbs after workout are the simplest. This includes pasta, rice potatoes, bread Oats, quinoa, quinoa and many more. Beware of white carbs and eat the whole grains.

Exception. If you're a slim man and want to lose weight loss, eat carbs, make sure you exercise, and submit exercise. If you'd like, add more.

6. Consume healthy fats. Fats that are healthy and whole increase the loss of fat and improves well-being. In addition, they are satiating and digest slowly, and are affordable. Take healthy fats every meal, and stay clear of artificial Trans fats and margarine. Make sure you are balancing your intake of fats.

Saturated fats. Boom testosterone ranges. Nutritional cholesterol isn't tied by blood cholesterol. Real butter, whole eggs and beefs.

Monounsaturated fats. Help prevent heart disease and cancer. More olive oil that is virgin and olives, mixed nuts.

Polyunsaturated fat. Increase testosterone levels; increase sales of fats loss, lessen infections, fish oil, flax seeds on the floor and blended nuts.

7. Drink plenty of water. Training for strength causes sweating and water loss that can hinder muscle recovery. Consuming water helps prevent dehydration as well as starvation on basis that a full stomach could make you believe that you're hungry.

1 US gallon water/day. Take 1 cup water as the before you when you wake up and 2

cups after every meal, and sip water while you workout.

Try to drink tea that isn't experienced and water with lemon squeezed.

Don't worry about drinking too much water. A healthy diet, as suggested in this article will ensure that that you have enough electrolytes. If you don't do anything crazy like drinking 2 gallons of water within 10 minutes and then you'll be safe.

8. Consume whole foods 90 percent of the all the time.

Whole foods. Foods that are unprocessed, and not refined (or very delicate) foods that are closest to their natural country. Examples: fresh meat, fish, chicken, eggs, veggies, legumes, fruits, rice, oats, quinoa,

Processed ingredients. They typically contain trans-fats, sugars as well as corn syrup, nitrates sodium, and other chemical substances. Examples: bagels bars pizza, cereals sausages, cookies frozen food as well as diet Supplements ...

Eat a balanced diet ninety percent of the all the time. The effect result is not significant compared to eating healthy and nutritious meals. If you consume 6 times a day it is possible to eat four unhealthy meals during the week without guilt. Similar to alcohol and sweet drinks 10 percent of the time, it's good enough.

A typical eating plan.

Breakfast: eggs and fruits, oranges, and unseasoned tea

Snack: mixed nuts, pear

Lunch: tuna, roman lettuce, olives, olive oil

Snack: cottage-cheese with apple

Post-exercise: ground-round and quinoa, spinach and banana

Dinner: fowl, spinach, toddler carrots, pear

Breakfast before bed Breakfast: cottage cheese, fruit, ground flax seeds and fish oil

Eating right

If you decide to try a weight lifting program, the food you consume can affect the efficacy of your training.

Many people don't pay careful attention to the kinds of food they consume.

However food is a vital element when it comes to lifting weights.

The food we eat provides us with calories. Calories are small amounts of energy your body needs to do tasks.

The importance of weighing calories is in it is determining which calories will be the most effective to get the maximum effect on your exercise.

To be able to perform your workout You'll need a range of supplements. The most important is sugars.

Chapter 11: Vegan Bodybuilding Mistakes

This is an overview of the most common mistakes that vegan bodybuilders should avoid, especially in order to keep building muscles without suffering an injury while doing it. Be sure to eliminate the mistakes and you will see a significant improvement in your progress!

1. Not paying attention to your body

You're getting ready for a trip to the gym for a chest exercise today however, your triceps and front delts are still sore after your shoulder workout the night before. You also got no sleep at all and feel extremely exhausted. What do you do?

Many bodybuilders with experience opt to exercise regardless. They adhere to the ethos of persevering through tough times, which is a great practice to adhere to, up to a certain extent. After a certain point however, you're just adding abuse over abuse.

It is important to pay attention to the body's signals or begs your to accomplish. It could be that it's signaling that you're in need of an hour or two of pure rest.

Perhaps it's telling you that trying to hit the next level in your skills every day isn't the most effective approach as a regular plan is better for your capabilities and lifestyle.

The athletes are constantly learning and growing. That's the only way to stay safe from injury. In the majority of cases, overtraining results in strains, tears and muscle tears. This could cause muscle loss and also time. Keep in mind that the short-term term isn't important when you're trying to build muscles!

Second error: Not training enough

In order to increase muscle size and strength You must challenge your muscles beyond what they are used to. The farther you push the greater.

You must perform each exercise until exhausted to keep your posture, using the weights you can lift to allow you to complete 10 or 20 slow and steady repetitions (by slow I mean you should need to take about 3 seconds for lifting the weight and another three seconds to lower the weight). You should also switch direction between lower and pumping movements without jerking, bumping or pulling the weight.

Don't stop the workout at the point that your muscles begin to swell or you feel slightly uncomfortable. This is when the most beneficial work has finished It's the highest point of your exercise. In the final few and most challenging repetitions, you'll get the best stimulus for building the strength of your muscles and their size. If you give into this position at the high point it is unlikely that you'll receive the same stimulation for growth.

3. Mistake A bad piece of advice

It is easy to be deceived in the present. We live in a time filled with information and therefore the best way to prevent this from happening is knowing which information is trustworthy. So, how do you find credible information from a reputable nutritionist/bodybuilder? An abs set? A contest trophy?

These things may appear to be a great proof however, when you think about the role of gene-based traits and also the unpublicized steroid a large portion of the people are taking in the business to get the amazing results, regardless, and even when they followed a weak program.

This could be very misleading for the novice or person who hasn't eating a hypocaloric diet for a long duration of. The idea that "their excellent shape is in line to what they're selling" can cause an unintentional confirmation bias for beginners and lead them to take an untrue path.

The truth is that the majority of people who show off their abs with six packs can't give you the amount of protein is needed to build muscle and thus aren't competent to give tips on your most precious asset your health.

4. Mistake 4: Switching routines or exercises frequently

The biggest gains can be achieved through continual progress on the most basic exercise over a long amount of time. The constant switching of routines hinders your body from getting over the initial audiovisual/skill adjustment stage, and, later the more important training that will follow.

The idea that you should be constantly changing your routine to avoid highs since our muscles are resistant to further development after specific exercises is due to the most rapid changes in your performance during the exercise program occur during the initial 6-8 weeks. Then , the performance slows down, and changing the regimen eventually solves the issue.

As mentioned earlier, in the first stages of performing the exercise for the first time more changes in the exercise are due to adaptations in the audiovisual or skill. After the initial period of audiovisual adaptation in the brain and performance, the overall level of performance starts to decline, and most of the adaption begins to take place in your muscles. This is the place where the most advancement is made it is vital to keep to your routine in this stage. The pace of progress will be slower than what it was during the first 6--8 weeks but it will help you to adjust to the frequency and volume of your workouts.

Contrary to common misconceptions about bodybuilding the muscles of your body do not cease to adjust to an workout, routine or procedure - however, in the event that a muscle is being over-worked and it begins to develop and when your intensity and frequency remain under control and you get adequate rest and food the muscles will grow and become stronger.

Fitness exercises for beginners to build muscle

There's no question about it: Bodybuilding can be an overwhelming task. If you're just beginning your journey to bodybuilding you must start with the right attitude to avoid burning out over the long run. Many hopeful bodybuilders start with programs that are too demanding for what they're used to and end up with failure and burning out.

An excellent program that employs simple techniques can help beginners in building an important muscles mass and fundamental strength. The amount of days you must train and the interval between them will be depending on the schedule you follow. It is recommended to begin with a simple, easy all-body routine every other day.

The plan includes a wide range of fundamental exercises that target the whole body during the exercise routine. The exercises must be ongoing and each one should differ from the previous. If you are a beginner exercise routine, these suggestions combined with a balanced diet such as the one in this book will give the best results in just only a couple of months.

The program is comprised of the following components:

Workout 1

3 sets of bench press, each comprising 10 reps

3 sets of squats of 10 reps

3 sets of crunches to do 20 reps

Deadlifts 3 sets, 10 reps

Workout 2

Bench press inline using dumbbells to perform 3 sets of 10 reps

Shoulder press overhead using dumbbells and 3 sets of reps

3 rows of barbells set in a row of 10 reps

3 sets stiff legged deadlift for 10 reps

3 sets of calf raises. 15 reps

3 sets leg presses for 10 reps

Workout 3

3 set of benches for 10 repetitions

3 set barbell curls for 10 reps

3 set leg extension for 10 repetitions

3 sets of frontal pull-downs for 10 reps

3 sets of crunches for 20 reps

A weekly breakdown of these exercises would look something like this:

Monday: First workout

Tuesday: First day of rest

Wednesday: Second session

Thursday: Second day of relaxation

Friday 3rd training session

Weekend: Relax days

This is a great option for novice bodybuilders. However, as the difficulties increase and you get comfortable with more weight lifting and a more demanding lifestyle, you'll need to schedule more time between muscles. If your schedule allows for the addition of a workout day each week, consider dividing your workouts into upper and lower the body splits.

This allows you to focus your focus on each workout and add some leisure time between the various of the body workouts so that every workout will be a bit more difficult.

Here's an example of how it might appear to be:

3 inclined bench presses of 10 reps

3 sets of pectoral flies of 10 reps

3 sets of pullups, each of which is 10 reps

3 sets of military press of 10 reps

3 sets deadlifts of 10 reps

3 sets of barbell curls of 10 reps

3 sets of crunches with 20 reps

Tuesday:

3 sets of squats, 10 reps

3 sets of leg curls, each with 10 reps

3 sets leg presses of 10 reps

3 sets of calf raises, each of 15 reps

3 sets of leg raises, each with 20 reps

Wednesday

Relax

Thursday

Repetition of Monday

Friday

(A repeat of Tuesday)

Saturday and Sunday

Relax

Whatever method you decide to follow regardless of the method you choose, it is essential to warm-up and stretch whatever prior to beginning the workout. This is to help ensure that blood circulation is flowing and the body stays in good shape for your exercise. Additionally, every exercise should be followed by a minimum of 20 minutes of cardiovascular exercise to help prevent injuries.

Begin with the basics. Don't overdo the isolation exercises. Instead, focus on multi-joint fusion exercises. The ideal routine for beginners needs to be followed during the initial up to 10 weeks to allow enough period of time to allow the body adjust to the workouts and build an established base in strength as well as mass. When that's done the workouts can be changed and the order of workouts altered.

Combine these exercises along with our diet and hydration program to feel fantastic, gain the energy you've never had before, and achieve the most out that you can ever make in the course of your lifetime!

Keep hydrated

When temperatures are high drinking enough water is vital, regardless of whether you're active in your sport or simply lying on the beach enjoying the sun.

Drinking a glass of water prior to a early morning workout, or sweating heavily during your workout, and having to endure extreme heat are all sure ways to dehydrate yourself. Drinking water when exercise can help in fighting fatigue and increase your endurance. Here are a few ways to check if you're properly hydrated. They are simple and easy to adhere to.

Urine color

The color of your urine can be an indicator of. If it's a clear colour, then the chance that you're well-hydrated is extremely high. In the event that the urine color appears dark, or has a peculiar smell, that's an indication that you are dehydrated. Be aware that if you are taking the B12 supplementation, this could influence the color of your urine. However, it doesn't mean that you're dehydrated. always consult your physician to find out what's happening if you're concerned about anything.

Rate of sweat

Another method of determining the level of hydration is to determine your weight prior to and following exercising. The weight difference between before and after you hydrate will give you an indication of your hydration levels. If you've added or retained exactly the same amount of weight it's possible to think that you're well-hydrated. If you're down in weight by a significant amount, you'll have to drink more water in order to recover the weight you've lost.

What is the recommended amount of water you should drink?

How much water need to drink varies; a person who sweats a lot is required to drink more than those who don't. This is particularly relevant for athletes who train in the scorching summer seasons. For every pound sweat that you shed, that's one pint of water that you need to replenish that's the reason it's not uncommon to see an athlete from a high school football team wearing pad and drills for running to shed 5 pounds of sweat training during the summer months.

Develop a habit of hydration

Many people work so hard to the point that they have no time to eat or even take a regular water break. However, a routine of drinking water will assist you to maintain your focus and energy levels so that your body and mind can function optimally. Here are some suggestions to make drinking fluids throughout the day.

Always carry water with you even when you're working.

Keep a water bottle in your bag It will be easier to drink drinking water all day long without feeling to be a hassle. If you feel tired or nauseous take a sip of cold water. It's an easy method to keep you alert whenever you're in an euphoria.

Consume a lot of whole foods

The water content of whole foods is naturally present and will dramatically boost the amount of fluid in your body in comparison to processed foods that contain very little or no water, leaving you exhausted and dehydrated.

Mix it up

Does the sound of water make you feel bored? Here are some suggestions to help you find different sources of water.

Mix it

Cut slices of fruit like limes citrus, lemons, and oranges in a glass container with water, and allow to cool for a couple of hours.

Mix in coconut Ice cubes

Incorporate the coconut water in your ice cube tray then pour the ice cubes into the glass of water to get the sweet and nutty flavor.

Sip herbal tea

Drink a cup of herbal tea each day. If you regularly do this and regularly, you'll add fluids from one cup of water added to your daily tally. In addition, this could be a great method to release tension at the end of the day.

Eat rice

Rice has super absorbent ingredients that work as a potent tool for replenishing your liquids after it's was cooked with water. Additionally, it has the advantage of boosting energy levels through carbohydrates. Beware of excessively salty rice dishes since excess sodium can hold water and can cause you to feel tired and bloated.

Drink up your water!

Try these food items to enjoy a tasty and easy method to increase the absorption of H20 without drinking water.

1 medium apple = 6 ounces

1 . Cup of watermelon ball

1 navel orange equals 4 1 ounces

1 cup of uncooked broccoli florets equals 2 8 ounces

1 cup cooked chopped zucchini = 6 ounces

1 Cup chopped, chopped Cantaloupe is 5 Ounces

10 baby carrots equals 3 1 ounces

If you don't sweat during intense exercise, it is a sign you're dehydrated to the extent of exhaustion because of the heat. You should also be wary of drinks with sugar as well as soda and fruit juices because they are harmful to your stomach, when you're not properly hydrated. Also, it is recommended to avoid drinking drinks made up of caffeine, as they may act as a diuretic, resulting to the loss fluids.

If you've a good understanding of the impact that drinking water can have on you, there is no need to fret for drinking more than 11 cups of water a every day as a routine.

Chapter 12: Bodybuilding For Beginners

Bodybuilding is a kind of resistance exercise that gradually builds up strength and helps you strengthen muscles. Anyone who is involved in this kind of exercise is known as an bodybuilder. Bodybuilding is a form of sport which requires a lot of discipline from the bodybuilder. When you are well-controlled, you remain consistently doing what you do by adhering to a workout plan. Bodybuilders who are disciplined do not flinch when they train; they keep exercising regardless of weather conditions, exhausted or not. They make sure they're eating right. If you are looking to get to the level of professional bodybuilding, you must work intensely and work more intensely.

How to begin bodybuilding

If you're serious about improving your fitness but aren't sure where to begin, here are a few suggestions that will help particularly if you're just starting to explore the fitness thing. These are tips that you can integrate into your routine. You can inquire for more information, read more, or conduct research and try various methods. Before you begin, obtain an approval from your physician.

1. Join a gym hunt

Find a location in which you will exercise the most exercise and bodybuilding. Find a gym that's clean and is equipped with the latest equipment. Another thing to consider is the presence of knowledgeable personnel and trainers. To ensure that you do not miss the gym, locate an area that is close to the location of your residence or workplace.

2. Set real-world goals

Make goals you can attain after a specified period of time. It is important to have realistic goals as unrealistic ones could leave you feeling disappointed at the final. Begin with small. Set realistic, short goals that you can achieve at the pace you prefer.

The primary goal you'd like to accomplish is to increase muscle strength and mass your body. After you have built up muscles that are strong and are ready to begin building your muscles.

When you plan to reach your goals, tackle them with the correct mindset. Perseverance and patience will aid you achieve your goals.

3. Be attentive to your body

Pay attention to the body's messages to convey to your body. If you're not in the mood Not because you're feeling tired, but rather because you feel unwell or sick, stop your workout and return to the gym once you feel much better.

Being unable to exercise in case you're sick is pointless.

4. Find a trustworthy trainer

It's helpful to have a trustworthy training partner when looking to gain muscle mass or enter the world of professional bodybuilding. Your training partner will be beneficial to you in achieving your goal of bodybuilding. With a buddy at training, it will be healthy competition since everyone will be more competitive, and your gains will be more rapid.

5. Stretching

Before beginning your workout, ensure that you stretch and warm your muscles in order to get the blood flowing. Begin with a light workout and stretch out the muscles you'll be training to work on that day.

6. Proper Breathing

A common bodybuilding and weightlifting method requires proper breathing, as it provides oxygen to your muscles . It is crucial for both contraction and growth.

How to do it When lifting, exhale and inhale when it lowers the weight.

7. Bodybuilding for beginners

Beginners need help on how to begin the process of bodybuilding.

8. Train on cycles

If you're a beginner and are just beginning, then you're probably thinking about how often you should exercise each muscle group. The rule of thumb is to rest for 48 hours prior to training the same muscle. In this way, you'll build up training routines.

Remember to take a break to relax your body.

9. Proper diet

You'll be able to lift the weights to the max However, you should keep a regular diet. If you don't, you won't get the results you'd like to achieve. It is crucial to ensure an appropriate diet that includes the correct quantity of calories from various food groups: proteins, fats and carbohydrates. Minerals and vitamins are crucial.

Every person will have a different approach to the way they eat based on their health and weight goals. In general, it is recommended to eat small portions, and to eat regularly instead of eating a large meal. Make sure you drink plenty of water.

10. Perform sets and repetitions of different exercises.

It is necessary to complete different sets and repetitions of various exercises. The repetitions indicate the amount of times you complete the exercises in succession. Likewise, sets are the blocks of repetitions for a particular exercise.

For instance, if you perform 3 sets with 15 reps for the push-up which is a push up, you must complete three sets of 15 push-ups in one row.

11. Combine cardio and aerobics

Once you've mastered the art of bodybuilding, and the fundamentals of weightlifting, do two or three cardio sessions every week to lose weight, maintain an active heart and reduce anxiety.

12. Supplements

You can boost your chances of achieving muscle mass by using protein powders.

This is highly recommended to beginner athletes to help them gain the lean mass of their muscles. Protein shakes are great option for between meals.

13. Relaxation and rest

After a long and intense workout the body needs to recover. Be sure to get an adequate night's sleep and don't overdo the exercise or other physical actions. The time between rest and exercise is when your muscles take in the proteins from your diet to help build their.

14. Training log

Track your progress in bodybuilding and keep a log of your workouts. Note down your training regimen along with the sets and reps you performed during your exercise. This will give you something to be looking forward to and keep track of your performance.

Chapter 13: How Often Each Body Part Is Trained

The goal should be to work out each part of your body every week for a minimum of one hour.

The growth of muscles occurs following the exercise. It takes a few days. If you are trying to train each muscle over and over the muscles won't be able to grow enough. This is usually the reason you'll feel weaker at the next exercise. It's due to the lack of time to complete the workout.

How many sets?

The first two sets of repetitions are an exercise to warming up.

If you decide to jump straight into using large weights, you could risk injury. If your muscles are cold they are more prone to tear. Therefore, by doing at least two warm-up exercises first, you can be able to avoid injuries.

The best method to build muscle is to begin with light weights. Gradually increase the weight for each exercise. This way your muscles will get prepared for the work sets.

The biggest mistake that people make when using this form or pyramid-training is not doing enough repetitions. The typical approach is to begin with light weights and then do as many repetitions as they can. This is a way to wear out muscles prior to the major sets. It is important to get your muscles prepared for the sets. It is not a good idea to become exhausted.

This is why you must do. It is recommended to do at least six repetitions. If you begin with a lighter set, it's going to feel effortless. As you get the weights heavier, the muscles will begin to warm up.

Make sure that the weight is increased in order that by the end of your third and fourth sets you'll have reached the weight of six repetitions. As an example, you'll remember that the last time, your 6 repetition weight was 200 pounds. It is possible to do six repetitions using 135 pounds. Then, you could do you could do a set of the equivalent of one hundred eighty pounds the third set of 200 pounds.

When you are at the point in the stage that you believe you are able to only complete six repetitions while maintaining good form, complete two sets of identical weight. It is likely that you are unable to finish six repetitions on the final set. This is because the muscles will be exhausted. Your final set will always be when you aren't able to complete six repetitions with proper form and control.

To summarise...

Perform two to three warm-up sets with heavier weights. Limit yourself to six repetitions per set. This will allow the muscles to warm up and not exhaust them.

If you reach the weight at which you can only complete six repetitions then continue to work with the same weight until six repetitions aren't possible.

Always ensure you have perfect form and control, and make sure that you are exercising throughout the entire range of your movements.

Rest between sets

Your muscles must take a break before you start the next workout. If you are too long, the muscle will begin to cool. Shorter and muscles may be exhausted. The ideal amount of time is 1 minute. This is the perfect amount of time.

Perfect shape

I was reading a book years ago that was called Flawless. It was written by Bob Paris. If you're not sure who you are, he's an bodybuilder who has a well-balanced body, with perfect symmetry. What is his secret?

He realized that a perfect shape led to an ideal body. His entire work stressed the importance of this.

As I mentioned previously the muscles have already got the ideal shape and size potential. They're just waiting to develop fully. (Fully inflated, just like balloons.)

What is the perfect shape?

Form is the art of moving the muscles on the direction they were designed to move in.

It also involves performing movements with the full range of motion. This is a reference to stretching from full to full contraction starting from the bottom and up to the top. In this way, the muscles will fully develop.

While your muscles perform the exercise, various parts will be in play. For example, at beginning of a curl with a barbell the lower portion of the biceps muscle is going to be employed. About halfway to the top, however, the middle part of the muscle will come into the game. So, if you do not make use of the full flexibility, you'll be missing out on certain areas of the muscle that are which are being trained. The muscle won't get into its most optimal form.

Take note of the balloon illustration earlier. If the muscle is the muscle is fully formed (inflated) muscles will appear in its most supple and slender.

I was able to do different exercises to strengthen my Biceps. However, in the end I discovered it was the use of a barbell that produced the greatest results. Many of my classmates began to praise the complete development of my Biceps. They noted that the muscles were developed all the way to my elbow.

The secret to success was that I made use of the entire range of motion. I would begin with my arms fully extended, then bring the weight upwards and downwards. This means it was built throughout its entire length. Always work to the fullest extent.

Position

It is also crucial to consider your posture. If your hands aren't wide enough or close together to each other, your muscle won't be fully trained. For instance, if you did a press with hands that are too close it would be more focus focused on the triceps, and less weight would be given to chest muscles.

Speed

In the event that you had to drive a vehicle it will be difficult the first time you started. Once the car was moving , it would become simpler. This is due to momentum. When the momentum is already in motion it's just a matter of maintaining it. It doesn't require you to exert as much effort.

If you are performing your repetitions You must ensure that your muscles are working throughout the workout. So, it is important to reduce the speed to an absolute minimum. It is achieved by maintaining the speed of your movement lower.

What I suggest is taking three seconds to lift the weight, and then three seconds to lower it. One thousand and one three, 12,000 and 2 one thousand three. It will take around three seconds.

Maintain the pressure on the muscles throughout the entire exercise. Be sure to not pause between the top and at the bottom of the set. If you stop then you'll take away the muscle's pressure and reduce the impact.

Symmetry and Shape

Utilizing barbells will provide you with the most effective results. I came across this information some time long time ago.

I would try various machines as well as dumbbell workouts. It wasn't until I began using barbells that my best results started to appear.

The reason behind this is because muscles are working equally across both sides of the body. This means that you build all of your muscles in a symmetrical way. Your body will look more attractive because of it.

Also, a way to boost your overall development is doing compound exercises. This means, exercises that work multiple muscles simultaneously.

The body prefers to work in a group. This is how the muscle system of the body is constructed. Muscles weren't designed to work as a unit.

Imagine picking up something that is heavy. If you stand up you will have several muscles engaged at the same time. It is likely that you'll be working your biceps, back, shoulder leg muscles, and back. All of them work together.

Another way to keep your body in balance by using the compound exercise. They are exercises that utilize multiple muscles at the same simultaneously. If you are doing compound exercises the muscles are built in proportion to one their counterparts.

I also noticed that I began getting stronger after I switched to compound exercises.

Isolation exercises like dumbbell raises lateral as well as smith machine presses leg machine extensions, did not yield any outcomes at all. These kinds of exercises are commonly called shaping exercises.

As previously mentioned, the muscles have a predefined shape. They will display their true shape once they have fully developed. The best method to accomplish this is with bars and compounds exercises.

There are some exceptions in this guarantee. The exceptions include chin-ups as well as crunches. But, chin-ups require the use of a bar. This time, however you are able to pull yourself to it. It's recommended to do your workout with your chin up bar.

Lat machines will not produce the identical results. This is due to the fact that you're pulling in the manner the machine was designed. When you chin-up the entire machine pulls naturally.

Exercises like crunches help to build abdominal muscles with just your own body weight. It is best not to train the pelvic muscles using weights. This is because weights can over-develop the pelvic region.

The abdominal muscles are best exercised with a crunching kind of motion. This is basically the way these muscles work. There are two types of muscles that are the most effective, and both will be discussed later.

A commonality is found in the exercises. This is because they are all common exercises. They bring a set of muscles. Like we said earlier, muscles are designed to collaborate. Training in this way improves the body's symmetry all over and promotes the highest growth.

How about curls of the bicep?

Biceps curls can be beneficial to build the full range of the muscles so long as they're done with the full range of motion.

There's no additional exercise to strengthen the biceps. What's the reason? Because these muscles are tiny in comparison to the larger muscles. This means that they are able to easily become over-trained.

The thing you must be aware of is that your biceps receive a workout when you perform other exercises that require pulling. For instance the biceps are utilized when doing the chin-up.

This is the same for trigeps, which are the three muscles in the rear in the arms. They only require one triceps exercise with the barbell. They also will benefit by doing all pushing exercises, like shoulders press and bench presses and so on.

Conclusion

Some believe that bodybuilding isn't meant for everyone however, I am not so sure. If you've started your own personal fitness program you will see that it's probably the most beneficial thing you've ever done to yourself. Not only will you appear better, but you'll be a confident person who wants to be the best in all areas of life. Regular exercise on a daily routine will improve your physical and mental health.

Nowadays, the majority of people want to lose weight by bodybuilding. If this is what drives you, then great. But, it is important to be aware of the benefits of working your body to complete exercises. When you've got that picture in your mind, you'll be able to see that there's many things you can learn from fitness.

There are countless examples from the past (and present) instances of individuals who have changed their lives due to bodybuilding. I provided two cases from ArnoldSchwarzenegger as well as Eugen Sandow at the start in this article. The outcomes they attain are not impossible, particularly for those willing to invest the time and effort required to accomplish such feats.

It does require lots of commitment and effort. But, keep in mind that the first step is the most challenging. Once you've completed the initial phase, you'll find that you're eager to keep exercising! In addition, you'll have that extra boost of motivation when you see your reflection and observe how you've done with your efforts.

What are you sitting on? Start immediately. Once you've figured out what you have to do and how to make your dream body an actual reality!

www.ingramcontent.com/pod-product-compliance
Lightning Source LLC
Chambersburg PA
CBHW071840080526
44589CB00012B/1065